Appetite In Training
My Journey to a Thinner Me

John M. Avery

"Nothing in the human realm can satisfy the soul, quite like the feeling of being light and agile."

CONTENTS

John M. Avery

Looking back and taking stock

"Time for a change."

The year was 2013. I had hit a high of two hundred and eighty seven pounds, the most I had ever weighed. As I looked at the scales, just thirteen pounds away from the three hundred pound mark, I said to myself, this is totally unacceptable.

I was tired of trying to pull my stomach in when out in public. I hated wearing a tie because I disliked the way it looked draped over a protruding mid-section. I was miserable. I felt like everyone was secretly judging me, although that was not the case. It was me judging me, and you know as well as I do that you are your own worst critic. But that was a good thing, because after having my fill of frustration, I was finally able to be honest with myself, and do something about the situation.

Engaging my retro vision, I remembered how I loved to eat. I had been raised on typical Southern fare, just good home cooking, however I had been active enough as a boy to avoid putting on too many excess pounds; stayed an acceptable weight for my height for the times. There was no talk of body mass index in those days. My ratio would have probably been unacceptable by today's standards, but I did alright in my world. I had a bicycle; rode quite a bit, and walked to school, two city blocks from home.

I remembered the Sunday lunches at my Grandma and Grandpa's house, things like stewed beef, mashed potatoes, gravy, homemade bread, green beans, and banana pudding for dessert. There was always enough left over to eat again in the evening. She usually cooked only twice on Sunday, breakfast and lunch.

Grandma had a philosophy she shared with me once. I never forgot it. Don't live to eat but eat to live, and I can say I never saw her overeat or overweight. I knew her words rang true, but at a young age, I looked forward to my next meal, because teenage boys as you know are eating machines.

On Friday evenings at my Grandparents' house we usually had a fish fry with all the fixings. It was not a religious tradition. We just loved seafood. The Friday evening fare was Fish, French fries, hushpuppies, coleslaw and a pot of oyster stew. Black coffee and Oreos was dessert.

Every year on Thanksgiving we had turkey, stuffing,

giblet gravy, cranberry sauce, green beans, and corn.

Our yearly Christmas meal was ham, potato salad, rolls, and all the little extras of the holiday, like a cheese ball, and various desserts.

Then there were the warm weather cookouts. I developed a very hearty appetite. I loved sour cream with salty potato chips and sour pickles, especially when we had cheeseburgers. In essence I loved all things that jazzed the taste buds. I had a taste for Mexican food; loved hot and spicy.

Through it all, I survived and remained in good health. However, I programed myself to eat big which meant having seconds and sometimes third servings of a particular item I really liked. I ate until I was just over full. When my parents took my siblings and me to an all you can eat seafood restaurant, I left stuffed.

Fortunately and unbelievably I arrived at adulthood at one hundred and eighty pounds; pretty slim for my height, because I was developing a habit that whenever I began getting thick in the midsection, I would cut back a bit, and sometimes fast a meal or two. Over the years though, I gradually worked my way upward to the two hundred and fifties. I thought I carried that well. At least it seemed so because of my six foot two inch frame, but I always knew I'd feel better being lighter.

Hard work, it seemed, had been my lot in life. I spent a lot of energy for a paycheck, so I made up for it at the table. I labored hard, doing everything from farm work to factory work, so I ate well. The idea, you'll work it off seemed to be working for me, as I was staying in the two hundred and forty and two hundred and fifty range, however, an early retirement brought an end to being able to eat big. I had to adjust my calories to fit my activities.

With the metabolism less efficient, and no everyday job, I ran the risk of putting on too many pounds. Even all the walking I was doing, three to four miles a day, and the yard work including push mowing could not negate the effects of having second and sometimes third helpings of my favorites at the table. I had a man sized appetite and it was high time as they say to put my appetite in training.

Getting Started

"A Time to Lose Weight; It isn't too late."

Plan A

My first plan of action was to eat no more than two thousand calories per day and keep up the walking. My walking these days is done mostly inside the house. The floor plan is such that I can walk through four of our rooms in a large oval, eighty feet multiplied by eighty feet equaling sixty four hundred feet, slightly over a mile.

On two thousand calories a day, the weight reduction was slow and if I had a weekend where eating out was either chosen or a thing of necessity then I regained some or all of what I had lost that week. The secret ingredient in restaurant foods I discovered was sodium. That's why it tastes so good, and what that salt did for me, of course, was keep me full of water while I packed on the fat. That's a double bloat.

Plan B

My second course of action was to eat extremely low carbohydrate, the result of a book we had bought. After doing it I would not recommend it. I didn't eat rice, potatoes, bread, most fruit, and some vegetables. I felt like trash but the pounds came off like magic. After several weeks on this diet I began to experience feelings of anxiety and had a couple panic attacks.

I suspect I was depleting my GABA reserves by not having any grains. I found that in my case, man shall not live on lean meat and greens alone. That was the end of the extreme low carbohydrate diet for me.

Plan C

Next I decided to eat a regular diet and keep it very healthy; get all my servings of grains, dairy, vegetables, fruits, nuts, protein, everything the body needed in proper amounts for maximum health, again the result of buying a book. I felt tremendous but started gaining weight. It became evident that I would not be able to eat everything suggested in this plan. I would be healthy and overweight. What a combination. Eventually the weight would cancel out the good effects of the food.

Three Strikes, You're out? Don't Think So

"No, Life isn't a ball game."

"Struck out? No, I don't think so. I'll choose another plan. I've already decided on an outcome which is a slim me so the world around me will have to come into alignment with my will; argument ended."

The Math Diet

"One, two, three; count that calorie."

After plan C, I began what I knew would work; the Math Diet; laugh out loud, simple addition; counting the calories. I started bumping the calories down gradually.

First I set myself a limit of fifteen to seventeen hundred per day then thirteen to fourteen, a gradual reduction.

Finally after several weeks I had worked my way down to one thousand to twelve hundred calories per day. My stomach was shrinking; couldn't hold large amounts of food. At one thousand calories, I'd usually lose one pound per day. At twelve hundred, I could lose a pound, or possibly stay the same. There were factors to consider like water intake, amount of activity and my body's response. There is one important down side to mention here. With this small amount of food, the body becomes irregular and will not eliminate waste for days.

I found that I had to really be smart with food choices at a thousand calories per day; no room for junk with that kind of calorie limits.

If I wanted junk food, I'd take just a little bite of something and count it. I once cut a chocolate covered marshmallow pie in fourths and ate the thing over a period of one week.

Activity was a big factor. If I had a day I had to work hard, do the lawn or other stuff, I had to increase my calories to around seventeen hundred or more. I thought in terms of how much fuel I needed to run on.

I weighed every morning which is probably the wrong thing to do. I watched the pounds go up and down. I kept a chart and found that it took about a month and a half to reduce ten pounds usually because there was the occasional eating out episodes. Sodium played a large role. I could go up five to seven pounds in just a weekend. Of course, it was water gain from high sodium food, and I could lose that in a short period of time. **The one thousand calorie a day diet was extremely difficult. I was hungry, and felt weak most of the time. I can see from my experience that it is not a healthy plan. It is almost a fast. I came to the conclusion that there is definitely no way one can take in enough nourishment eating only one thousand to twelve hundred calories per day.**

As a man I found this experimental diet extremely difficult. I could do no physical labor on this kind of calorie intake. I had been desperate to be rid of the excess weight. **However In retrospect, I have to say that I got in too big of a hurry with the weight loss. Sixteen to eighteen hundred calories a day would be a more sensible plan, and this is what I eventually had to do in order to lose weight and still remain healthy.**

Listen To Your Body

"Body speaks; be all ears."

As I dieted I had to learn how to pay attention to how I felt. I eventually could tell when I needed more protein, or more water, or even a little healthy sugar, like a small serving of honey. If you'll consider your feelings your body will talk to you. Know what your body needs and feed it, and very important, **everyone's metabolism is not the same. You may need more calories than someone else.** Also, protein is of the utmost importance, and not all protein is meat. The body is a biological machine. It needs proper fuel.

When counting calories it is best to count the largest meal of the day first which for most people is dinner. That way you can divide up what you have left between breakfast and lunch. These two meals can be divided equally if you choose, but most importantly start the day with a written plan of action, what you'll eat and how much.

Most experts will say, do not skip breakfast. I agree. A bit of protein and carbohydrate seems to get me off to a great start. Your breakfast can be anything you choose as long as it fits into your calorie count. This is true for lunch and dinner. If you have chosen to go on eighteen hundred calories a day for example, you might have a three hundred calorie breakfast, a five hundred calorie lunch, and a thousand calorie dinner, and you may borrow calories from one meal or all to have a snack or snacks during the day.

You set your own limits, and when you are setting the limits, you are building emotional strength

Make Room for Junk Food

"Cut that snack cake into eight pieces and eat one piece."

Most of us love junk food, and some say avoid it, but I did not take that approach. If I wanted something, I just worked it into my calorie count for the day. Look at it this way. When you can eat just a bite of something and put it away for another day you are, as I referenced earlier, building emotional strength. You are not letting the food dictate how and what you eat. When you say no, can't have that, you are in a weird sort of way reinforcing the craving. Food is something we need in order to live, and while it is true we do not actually need the potato chips or the cookies, a limited amount will bring pleasure and do no harm.

Personally, I do not agree with using the word addiction in connection to food. It is true that people can lose control over how much and what they eat, being convinced that they need certain foods, but with small steps they can reprogram themselves to eat in a more sensible manner. Habits are formed with consistently repeated efforts.

Foods, like people have reputations of being good and bad, but if you can see all food as equal in value, the carrot and the cookie, refusing to judge one good or bad, you can deal with the craving. Rather see the value in benefits. Granted the carrot has more benefits than the cookie for health, but the cookie has benefits in satisfying a taste. You must decide what is more important to you. If you sacrifice health for the sake of satisfying a craving for sweets, like going crazy with dessert, you have a stumbling block in your way. The cookie being less valuable to your body than a carrot, is of course given a place of lower importance, therefore its serving size is minimal. Have a bite or eat just one; no need to abstain. Satisfying the taste for something sweet is not without value.

Being Determined

"No one can do for you what you should do yourself."

Making a healthy eating plan is not something you can do with your brain in neutral. It requires some thought and planning, reading labels and calculating values. It's much easier to order a number six at your favorite burger joint with large fries and a drink. The plan will get you where you want to be in time. The number six as a repetitive thing will keep you where you don't want to be. Remember, you are the architect and the builder of the house you live in. Will it be a house of health or shack of sickness?

No, fast foods are not the problem. The love of fast foods is the problem. When you love the pleasure the food brings you more than you love the body you live in then it is a problem. Love yourself enough to make a plan and let it jazz you. Keep the image of what you want to be in your mind. You may have setbacks. You may have to lose the same ten pounds over and over but eventually you'll get there if you don't quit.

Develop the ability to forgive yourself and go for it again. Nature's reward to you for losing pounds is that you began to feel the lightness right away, and when you begin to feel lighter you become inspired to lose more. So start creating those feelings through the power of imagination even though the excess is still there. Feel your way to inspiration.

Don't Grieve Over Food

"You have not lost a thing."

When attempting to eat less, I find that it is natural to experience a sense of grief over what you are not getting. Case in point is my famous peanut butter and jelly sandwich which I find impossible now to eat with my new standards being what they are, yet it lives on in my memory as the picture of what a peanut butter and jelly sandwich should be, and I often day dream about it. I may someday just eat one. After all, it's not likely I could pick up ten pounds from a single sandwich. Let me construct the image of my favorite sandwich for you. Start with two nice pieces of white bread, fresh and soft. Spread one side with peanut butter about one quarter inch thick, the other side with grape jelly, about half the measure of the peanut butter. Dust the jelly with lots of cinnamon, slap together and enjoy with a glass of very cold milk. This is all about taste and nothing more. It is quite possible that this meal was around eight hundred calories. I don't know. It certainly stayed with me awhile anyway. I made a half of a sandwich recently using minimal amounts of nut butter and jelly, and low calorie bread, a one hundred and sixty calorie version which I had with black coffee. Let me tell you; it was a big disappointment.

Nevertheless, I am jazzed with the numbers I'm seeing on the scales and am not ready to return to indiscriminate eating. If you don't measure your food, you do not know what you are putting in you, and at the end of the day you end up bloated and all weighted down. **I found that portion control was the only way to reduce and lose the unwanted pounds.**

How do you get past the false feeling of grief over not having all that you want? First you must understand that nothing has changed. You can still have whatever food you want and in any amount you want. It's just that you are at this moment choosing not to because you're after something better than jazzing your palate. You're after a leaner look, and a healthier body. Everything of value costs something.

Understanding Temptation

"Understand yourself."

Need for food is one of the strongest urges you have and for obvious reasons. You need food of course to live but you must develop an attitude that you don't need as much as you think you do. Appetite only knows two things: This is good and I want it. In order to train the appetite in a successful manner you must have the attitude that you may eat anything you want to eat, but you may not eat as much as you think you want. That's really what the problem is, thinking you want a lot of something. See yourself as someone who can be trusted to do the right thing; the right thing being to eat only what is necessary for strength and health. When you sit down to eat, see in your mind's eye, yourself as a slim person eating that meal. Begin to feel slim in your thoughts. As you walk imagine yourself feeling light on your feet. Create the feelings inside. The reality of it will show up on the outside eventually.

Don't Fear the Temptation

"You just have to take control."

Do not stress over the temptation; welcome it. For example, keep a bag of chips or a box of cookies purposely in plain view. Be convinced that you will not go crazy and eat too much; you will have a little when you can work it in to your plan. Be proud of the fact that the goodies are lasting long enough to go out of date. Don't be afraid of temptation. Temptation is an opportunity to show yourself strong. Appetite training as well as all good habits that one wishes to put in place is established best in the presence of temptation.

The key to overcoming the urge to eat too much is using serving sizes and seeing in your mind's eye yourself being rewarded with a thinner body for doing so.

Maintaining Where You Are

"Keep your goal in plain view before you."

March 2015; I am holding between 215 and 222 pounds. I still have a goal of reaching 200 lbs. I am finding in order to maintain where I am, I must stay in the mindset that got me to where I am. You cannot become lax, nor can you forget how miserable you were at your heaviest weight.

It is an easy thing to become content with reaching a portion of your goal and put its fulfillment off by pushing it further and further into the future. However, someday never happens upon the scene unless you through sheer determination make it do so. I will never go back to my heaviest weight, because I have settled that fact in my heart.

Setback

"It's only temporary."

May 2015, birthday celebration; a family cookout is in order, plus a few restaurant meals. Weight gain is inevitable, but not to worry, I'll engage a little maintenance in the way of cutting back, using some or all of the methods that helped me get to my lowest weight. It just takes a bit of time. The pounds did not come to stay. What I learned along the way will help me maintain. There was value in low carbohydrate eating. It was good for a jumpstart on my weight loss, but it was nothing I could do long term. A diet of meat, cheese, and salad is not exactly the healthiest fare to subsist on long term. However, one could resort to a high protein, low carbohydrate diet for a few days to get rid of a few pounds. Reality is though, that calorie awareness will come back into the picture. **Refuse to look at the calories on the menu and you'll look at them in the mirror.** Which is less painful?

Come Back

"No problem."

Fast forward; I'm back on track. It is summer, which is a good thing. There is yard work to do, and other activities, some actually fun. Activity is my friend and yours. Walking is one of the best ways to maintain a healthy weight. **A good brisk walk of one mile can burn around a hundred calories, and that is a real bargain.**

Add, Don't Take Away

"Remember to eat the sweets, but don't forget the best."

The secret to losing weight and keeping it off is not by abstaining from things, but rather adding to your diet. Doing totally without certain foods you love makes you want them all the more. It is for certain that you will lose weight by avoiding bread, potatoes, rice, pastries & sweets, etcetera, but there's another way, a healthier way. What if you continued to have just a little of the so called bad stuff, and added to it some healthy stuff; vegetables like, cabbage, broccoli, cauliflower, onions, bell peppers, celery, cucumbers, tomatoes, spinach, pumpkin, zucchini, carrots, green peas, squash, sweet potatoes, Brussels sprouts, lettuces? You get the picture; Broccoli with cheese sauce and bacon crumble, maybe? My point is that severely limiting what you can have causes you to feel deprived. This will eventually lead to binge eating. Have the occasional burger, or the pizza.

Health screams at us in vibrant colors, green spinach, yellow squash, orange carrots, red tomatoes, purple beets. Fruits and vegetables alike come in eye catching colors, designed by Nature's creator to get our attention, but we learn to look at them the way we do the wildflowers, pretty but uninteresting.

What we eat is for the most part is a product of tradition. We grow up with certain foods and that's basically what we eat all our lives. **Learn to make room for fruits and vegetables and you will be rewarded with a leaner and healthier body. Also add high fiber fruits and veggies. Don't depend just on grains for fiber. Above all drink clean natural water. Stay hydrated.**

Learn to research foods and find out their benefits for the body. Become your own nutritionist. Know what you need for optimal health. You will find that the healthier foods are a bit more expensive, but doctor visits are pricier.

Create Affirmations to Keep You Slim

"I am what I believe about myself."

If you can accept it, your words can change your reality. No, our words are not magic. We cannot say, I am slim and beautiful, or slim and handsome, whatever the case may be, and in the first three seconds be that. However, our words do get into our heart and play a big role in changing us.

Each one of us has a self-image that we carry around on the inside. It may not be apparent to others but we see it clearly. As in the case of weight, our heavy self is kind of hard to disguise on the outside. I wore a lot of black in an attempt to look smaller, and at one time would not tuck my shirt tail in. I was big, but not as big as the image I kept on the inside. I had to start seeing the person I was on the inside getting smaller before the man on the outside could make progress.

Of course food, or rather lack of food played a major role. I had to start eating less in order to reduce, but the weight loss could not have been initiated without the vision changing inside me. I had a vision inside me that said, I could not reduce any lower than two hundred and fifty pounds. If I did lose five or ten pounds, I would eventually go back up. It was like a thermostat set on two hundred and fifty. If I decreased in pounds, the belief would see to it that I got back up to my true identity, which was a two hundred and fifty pound man.

I once had a belief that I could not be satisfied, unless I had bread with my meals. I had to change that belief. I still eat bread, but usually only one piece of toast in the morning.

I once thought I had to clean out the pots. I now put food up for another day, or toss it out for a stray dog. I had to see myself doing these things, and being this way. Everything in my life is not ideal, but what I can change to suit my ideals, I do. My appetite was something I could change.

A word of caution; humor is something we must be careful with. Case in point, I would occasionally stuff a pillow under my shirt to get a few laughs, not realizing that I was portraying myself to myself as a heavier man.

We must watch our words as well. I would often say, "I'm as ravenous as a wolf, and I just can't get satisfied." Our words will cause us to feel a certain way. If we feel satisfied, we won't be looking for something more. If we feel dissatisfied, we will forage; go for a few crisps or crackers after a meal.

We have to set the stage for our success then follow the script. Be an actor in a movie portraying the person we want to be. A slim person is not grazing throughout the day. A slim person will eat a well- planned meal and be satisfied. A slim person will tend to be more active, have a spring in his or her step, and be more agile.

As we begin to have a vision inside us of becoming that slimmed down version of ourselves, creating affirmations will help. They will bolster our beliefs. A statement like, "I am grateful that I see the readout on the scales at my ideal weight, and I am thankful that I am slim, trim, and healthy," will move you in the direction of your goal. A statement like, "It is so hard to lose weight," will actually impede your progress. Talk to the Universe; make your intentions known. "I am," is a powerful affirmation. Whatever you put behind those words, whether good or bad, creates. Before a house is built, someone has to dream it, and talk about it then make a plan, and take action. It's the same with anything. If you are ever going to be your ideal weight, you'll have to dream it, declare it, plan it then take action.

Also of great importance are our feelings. They will move us toward or away from the attainment of any goal. Ask yourself, "How would I feel if I were slim?" then began to feel that way in your imagination. Keep that image of the new and improved you always in your thoughts. See yourself in the clothes you'd be wearing, and the activities you'd be engaged in. Feel like you are already that person. Realize that when you mentally choose the new you, that the current version of you is just a persistent illusion hiding a better image, an ideal picture. In time if you persist in holding the ideal reflection of you in your mind, it will appear. All things at your disposal will work together for good to bring your ideal into manifestation. Food in the right amount will work to that end. Exercise, water, sleep, determination, and belief will work to that end. Begin at this moment in time to be convinced in your heart, that you are the ideal version of yourself.

Good Luck

"I wish you much success in your weight loss journey."

"I hope my story has inspired and encouraged you. Never ever give up. You can be the person you want to be. And, remember to never stop loving you. You need the love and support of yourself as much as you need the love and support of family and friends."

Best Wishes, John M. Avery

Thank you for purchasing this book. I hope you were encouraged, and your thoughts expanded.

If you liked this book, please leave a review; it would be appreciated.

Please look for my other books. Below is an excerpt from a future book **"Appetite in Training II--Thin and Healthy"**:

Appetite in Training II--Thin and Healthy:

"In your weight loss journey you may find yourself stuck at a certain point on the scales. In order to break that pound barrier, you will have to make adjustments."

Keep informed of upcoming books by joining me on Facebook, Twitter, and don't forget the blog.

Blog: **https://johnmavery.wordpress.com**

Twitter: **https://twitter.com/JohnAvery7**

Facebook: **https://www.facebook.com/pages/John-M-Avery/166932053371986?ref=hl**

Email: **javery512@gmail.com**

www.ingramcontent.com/pod-product-compliance
Lightning Source LLC
Chambersburg PA
CBHW070935290526
45795CB00003B/1024